CW00586645

The Homemade Cookbook

Many fantastic DIY recipes, easy to make at home. More than 50 recipes for you and your family

(*VOL.1*)

Table Of Contents

Grandma's Homemade Banana Bread

Ingredients

1 1/2 cups white sugar
1/2 cup butter, softened
3 bananas, mashed
2 eggs
2 cups all-purpose flour
1/2 teaspoon baking soda
1/3 cup sour milk
1/4 teaspoon salt
1 teaspoon vanilla extract

Directions

Preheat oven to 350 degrees F (175 degrees C). Lightly grease an 8x4 inch loaf pan.

Combine sugar, butter, bananas, eggs, flour, baking soda, milk, salt and vanilla extract in a large mixing bowl; beat well. Pour batter into prepared pan.

Bake in a preheated oven for 60 minutes, or until a toothpick inserted into the center of the loaf comes out clean.

Homemade Vanilla

Ingredients

1 (750 milliliter) bottle vodka
2 vanilla beans

Directions

Submerge vanilla beans in vodka and store in a cool, dark place for several weeks, shaking occasionally.

Homemade Vegetable Soup

Ingredients

2 cups chopped baby carrots
2 baking potatoes, cut into cubes
1 small sweet onion, chopped
2 stalks celery, chopped
1 (14 ounce) can great Northern beans, rinsed and drained
1/2 small head cabbage, chopped
1 (14 ounce) can diced tomatoes
2 cups cut fresh green beans (1/2 inch pieces)
1 (32 ounce) carton chicken broth
2 (14 ounce) cans vegetable stock
2 cups water
1 1/2 teaspoons dried basil
1 pinch rubbed sage
1 pinch dried thyme leaves
salt to taste

Directions

Combine the baby carrots, potatoes, onion, celery, beans, cabbage, tomatoes, green beans, chicken broth, vegetable stock, water, basil, sage, thyme, and salt in a large pot; bring to a boil. Reduce heat to low; cover. Simmer until vegetables are tender, about 90 minutes.

Homemade Pancake Syrup

Ingredients

3/4 cup packed brown sugar
1/4 cup sugar
3/4 cup water
1/2 cup light corn syrup
1/2 teaspoon maple flavoring
1/2 teaspoon vanilla extract

Directions

In a saucepan, combine the sugars, water and corn syrup; bring to a boil over medium heat. Broil for 7 minutes or until slightly thickened. Remove from the heat; stir in maple flavoring and vanilla. Cool for 15 minutes. Serve over pancakes, waffles or French toast.

Homemade Peanut Butter Cups

Ingredients

2 cups milk chocolate chips
2 tablespoons shortening
1/2 cup butter
1/2 cup crunchy peanut butter
1 cup confectioners' sugar
2/3 cup graham cracker crumbs

Directions

In 1-quart saucepan combine chocolate chips and shortening. Cook over low heat, stirring occasionally, until melted and smooth (3 to 5 minutes).

Loosen top paper cup from stack, but leave in stack for greater stability while being coated. With small paint brush, coat inside top cup evenly with about 1 teaspoon melted chocolate to about 1/8-inch thickness, bringing coating almost to top of cup, but not over edge. Repeat until 30 cups are coated; refrigerate cups.

In 2-quart saucepan combine butter or margarine and peanut butter. Cook over medium heat, stirring occasionally, until melted (4 to 6 minutes). Stir in confectioners' sugar and graham cracker crumbs. Press about 1/2 tablespoon filling into each chocolate cup.

Spoon about 1/2 teaspoon melted chocolate on top of filling; spread to cover. Freeze until firm (about 2 hours) carefully peel off paper cups. Store refrigerated.

Homemade Fresh Pumpkin Pie

Ingredients

2 cups mashed, cooked pumpkin
1 (12 fluid ounce) can evaporated milk
2 eggs, beaten
3/4 cup packed brown sugar
1/2 teaspoon ground cinnamon
1/2 teaspoon ground ginger
1/2 teaspoon ground nutmeg
1/2 teaspoon salt

2 2/3 cups all-purpose flour
1 teaspoon salt
1 cup shortening
1/2 cup cold water

Directions

Preheat oven to 400 degrees F (200 degrees C).

Halve pumpkin and scoop out seeds and stringy portions. Cut pumpkin into chunks. In saucepan over medium heat, in 1 inch of boiling water heat the pumpkin to a boil. Reduce heat to low, cover and simmer for 30 minutes or until tender. Drain, cool and remove the peel.

Return pumpkin to the saucepan and mash with a potato masher. Drain well.

Prepare pie crusts by mixing together the flour and salt. Cut shortening into flour, add 1 tablespoon water to mixture at a time. Mix dough and repeat until dough is moist enough to hold together.

With lightly floured hands shape dough into a ball. On a lightly floured board roll dough out to 1/8 inch thickness. With a sharp knife, cut dough 1 1/2 inch larger than the upside down 8-9 inch pie pan. Gently roll the dough around the rolling pin and transfer it right side up on to the pie pan. Unroll, ease dough into the bottom of the pie pan.

In a large bowl with mixer speed on medium, beat pumpkin with evaporated milk, eggs, brown sugar, cinnamon, ginger, nutmeg and salt. Mix well. Pour into a prepared crust. Bake 40 minutes or until when a knife is inserted 1 inch from the edge comes out clean.

REAL Homemade Pumpkin Pie

Ingredients

1 medium sugar pumpkin
1 teaspoon ground nutmeg
1 teaspoon ground ginger
1 teaspoon salt
3 cups evaporated milk
4 eggs, beaten
2 (9 inch) unbaked pie crusts

Directions

Preheat oven to 400 degrees F (200 degrees C).

Cut out top of pumpkin and clean out all seeds and strings from inside. Slice pumpkin vertically into 3 inch wide strips. Place strips onto a baking sheet.

Bake in preheated oven for about 1 hour. Once done, scrape the pumpkin from the skins, then beat with a mixer or puree in a food processor until smooth.

Preheat oven to 425 degrees F (220 degrees C).

Mix the nutmeg, ginger, salt, evaporated milk and eggs with the pumpkin puree. Pour mixture into two 9 inch pie crusts.

Bake in preheated oven for 15 minutes. Reduce oven temperature to 350 degrees F (175 degrees C) and bake for an additional 35 to 40 minutes, or until toothpick inserted into center comes out clean. Cool and refrigerate.

Hayley's Homemade Lemon Cordial

Ingredients

2 cups white sugar
2 cups water
1 teaspoon lemon extract
1 1/2 teaspoons cream of tartar

Directions

In a saucepan combine sugar, water and cream of tartar. Heat until sugar is dissolved but don't boil. Remove from heat. Add lemon essence and let mixture cool.

Homemade Chicken Broth

Ingredients

2 1/2 pounds bony chicken pieces
2 celery ribs with leaves, cut into chunks
2 medium carrots, cut into chunks
2 medium onions, quartered
2 bay leaves
1/2 teaspoon dried rosemary, crushed
1/2 teaspoon dried thyme
8 whole peppercorns
2 quarts cold water

Directions

Place all ingredients in a soup kettle or Dutch oven. Slowly bring to a boil; reduce heat. Skim foam. Cover and simmer for 2 hours. Set chicken aside until cool enough to handle. Remove meat from bones. Discard bones; save meat for another use. Strain broth, discarding vegetables and seasonings. Refrigerate for 8 hours or overnight. Skim fat from surface.

Homemade Root Beer

Ingredients

6 cups white sugar
3 1/3 gallons cold water
1 (2 ounce) bottle root beer
extract
4 pounds dry ice

Directions

In a large cooler, mix together the sugar and water, stirring to dissolve sugar completely. Stir in the root beer extract. Carefully place the dry ice into the cooler, and cover loosely with the lid. Do not secure the lid, as pressure may build up.

Let the mixture brew for about an hour before serving. Leftover root beer can be stored in one gallon milk jugs.

Homemade Mashed Potatoes

Ingredients

5 medium baking potatoes, peeled and sliced
1 cup shredded Monterey Jack cheese
1/2 cup garlic seasoned bread crumbs
1/2 cup milk
1 tablespoon butter
salt and pepper to taste

Directions

Preheat the oven to 400 degrees F (200 degrees C).

Place the potatoes into a saucepan, and fill with enough water to cover. Bring to a boil. Cook for 5 to 10 minutes, just until soft. Drain water, and mash potatoes. Beat in the butter, and about half of the milk using an electric mixer. Add more milk if needed to achieve the desired consistency of mashed potato. Season with salt and pepper.

Spread potatoes evenly in a 9x13 inch baking dish, or desired casserole dish. Sprinkle the bread crumbs and cheese over the top.

Bake for about 10 minutes in the preheated oven, until the cheese is melted and the top is browned. Serve immediately.

Homemade Wine

Ingredients

1 (.25 ounce) package active dry yeast
4 cups sugar
1 (12 fluid ounce) can frozen juice concentrate - any flavor except citrus, thawed
3 1/2 quarts cold water, or as needed

Directions

Combine the yeast, sugar and juice concentrate in a gallon jug. Fill the jug the rest of the way with cold water. Rinse out a large balloon, and fit it over the opening of the jug. Secure the balloon with a rubber band.

Place jug in a cool dark place. Within a day you will notice the balloon starting to expand. As the sugar turns to alcohol the gasses released will fill up the balloon. When the balloon is deflated back to size the wine is ready to drink. It takes about 6 weeks total.

Homemade Egg Bread

Ingredients

2 (.25 ounce) packages active dry yeast
1/2 cup warm water (110 degrees F to 115 degrees F)
1 1/2 cups warm milk (110 to 115 degrees F)
1/4 cup sugar
1 tablespoon salt
3 eggs, beaten
1/4 cup butter, softened
7 cups all-purpose flour
1 egg yolk
2 tablespoons water
Sesame seeds

Directions

Dissolve yeast in water. Add milk, sugar, salt, eggs, butter and 3-1/2 cups flour; mix well. Stir in enough remaining flour to form a soft dough. On a floured surface, knead until smooth and elastic, 6-8 minutes. Place in greased bowl; turn once to grease top. Cover and let rise in warm place until doubled, 1-1/2 to 2 hours. Punch down. Cover and let rise until almost doubled, about 30 minutes. Divide into six portions. On a floured surface, shape each into a 14-in.-long rope. For each loaf, braid three ropes together on greased baking sheet; pinch ends to seal. Cover and let rise until doubled, about 50 to 60 minutes. Beat egg yolk and water; brush over loaves. Sprinkle with sesame seeds. Bake at 375 degrees F for 30-35 minutes.

Homemade Chicken Soup

Ingredients

1 (3 pound) whole chicken
4 carrots, halved
4 stalks celery, halved
1 large onion, halved
water to cover
salt and pepper to taste
1 teaspoon chicken bouillon
granules (optional)

Directions

Put the chicken, carrots, celery and onion in a large soup pot and cover with cold water. Heat and simmer, uncovered, until the chicken meat falls off of the bones (skim off foam every so often).

Take everything out of the pot. Strain the broth. Pick the meat off of the bones and chop the carrots, celery and onion. Season the broth with salt, pepper and chicken bouillon to taste, if desired. Return the chicken, carrots, celery and onion to the pot, stir together, and serve.

Homemade Tomato Sauce I

Ingredients

10 ripe tomatoes
2 tablespoons olive oil
2 tablespoons butter
1 onion, chopped
1 green bell pepper, chopped
2 carrots, chopped
4 cloves garlic, minced
1/4 cup chopped fresh basil 1/4
teaspoon Italian seasoning 1/4
cup Burgundy wine
1 bay leaf
2 stalks celery
2 tablespoons tomato paste

Directions

Bring a pot of water to a boil. Have ready a large bowl of iced
water. Plunge whole tomatoes in boiling water until skin starts to
peel, 1 minute. Remove with slotted spoon and place in ice bath.
Let rest until cool enough to handle, then remove peel and squeeze
out seeds. Chop 8 tomatoes and puree in blender or food
processor. Chop remaining two tomatoes and set aside.

In a large pot or Dutch oven over medium heat, cook onion, bell
pepper, carrot and garlic in oil and butter until onion starts to soften,
5 minutes. Pour in pureed tomatoes. Stir in chopped tomato, basil,
Italian seasoning and wine. Place bay leaf and whole celery stalks in
pot. Bring to a boil, then reduce heat to low, cover and simmer 2
hours. Stir in tomato paste and simmer an additional 2 hours.
Discard bay leaf and celery and serve.

Homemade Flaxseed Donuts

Ingredients

3 cups all-purpose flour
1/2 cup ground flaxseed
1 tablespoon baking powder
1/2 teaspoon ground nutmeg
1/2 teaspoon ground cinnamon
2 eggs
1 cup white sugar
1 cup buttermilk
2 tablespoons vegetable oil

1 quart vegetable oil for frying

Directions

Whisk the flour, flaxseed, baking powder, nutmeg, and cinnamon together in a bowl until evenly blended; set aside. Beat the eggs and sugar together in a separate bowl; whisk the buttermilk and 2 tablespoons of vegetable oil into the egg mixture. Stir the flour mixture into the egg mixture until no lumps of flour remain and the dough is firm enough to handle. Cover the bowl and refrigerate at least 10 minutes.

Roll the dough to 1/2-inch thickness on a generously-floured surface. Use a floured donut cutter to cut donut shapes out of the dough. Let the donuts stand for 5 to 10 minutes as the oil heats.

Heat the frying oil in a deep-fryer or large saucepan to 360 degrees F (180 degrees C).

Fry the donuts in the hot oil in batches until golden brown on both sides, about 2 minutes per side. Drain on a paper towel-lined plate before serving.

Homemade Vegetable Juice Cocktail

Ingredients

15 pounds fresh tomatoes
2 cups chopped celery
3 large onions, peeled and cut into chunks
1 green bell pepper, seeded and chopped
2 medium beets
4 carrots
3 cloves garlic, peeled
1/4 cup sugar
1 teaspoon black pepper
2 teaspoons prepared horseradish
1/3 cup lemon juice
6 quarts water, or as needed
1 tablespoon Worcestershire sauce, or to taste
1 cup white sugar
1/4 cup salt, or to taste

Directions

Use a juicer to process the tomatoes, celery, onion, green pepper, beets, carrots, and garlic. Place all of the juice into a large pot. Stir in the sugar, black pepper, horseradish, lemon juice, and enough water to make a thin consistency. Season with Worcestershire sauce to taste. Bring to a boil, and continue boiling for 20 minutes.

Ladle into 1 quart jars leaving 3/4 inch of headspace. Stir 1 tablespoon of sugar and 1 teaspoon of salt into each jar. Wipe rims clean, and place lids and rings onto jars. Process in a pressure canner for 35 minutes at 10 pounds of pressure.

Homemade Pork Sausage

Ingredients

2 pounds ground pork
2 teaspoons ground sage
1 1/2 teaspoons salt
1 1/2 teaspoons pepper
1/2 teaspoon cayenne pepper
1/2 teaspoon brown sugar

Directions

In a bowl, combine all ingredients; mix well. Shape into eight 4-in. patties. In a skillet over medium heat, fry patties for 3-4 minutes per side until browned or until no longer pink in the center.

Homemade Wonderful Bread

Ingredients

2 1/2 teaspoons active dry yeast
1/4 cup warm water (110 degrees F/45 degrees C)
1 tablespoon white sugar
4 cups all-purpose flour
1/4 cup dry potato flakes
1/4 cup dry milk powder
2 teaspoons salt
1/4 cup white sugar
2 tablespoons margarine
1 cup warm water (110 degrees F/45 degrees C)

Directions

Whisk together the yeast, 1/4 cup warm water and sugar. Allow to sit for 15 minutes.

Add ingredients in the order suggested by your manufacturer, including the yeast mixture. Select the basic and light crust setting.

Homemade Albondigas Soup

Ingredients

1 pound ground beef
1 bunch cilantro, finely chopped
1 small onion, chopped
4 cloves garlic, minced
1 pinch garlic salt
1 pinch onion powder
salt and ground black pepper to taste

4 (14.5 ounce) cans chicken broth
4 large carrots, cut into 1/2 inch pieces
3 stalks celery, cut into 1 inch pieces
3 potatoes, cubed

Directions

Place the ground beef, 1/2 of the cilantro, 1/2 of the chopped onion, the garlic, garlic salt, and onion powder in a bowl. Sprinkle with salt and black pepper, and mix gently until combined. Form the meat mixture into golf ball-sized meatballs.

Spray a large skillet with nonstick spray, and brown the meatballs carefully over medium-high heat; remove the meatballs and set aside (the meatballs do not need to be fully cooked; they will finish cooking in the soup). Cook and stir the remaining onion in the same skillet over medium-low heat until translucent, about 10 minutes.

Pour the chicken broth into a large pot, and stir in the onion; add the carrots, celery, and potatoes. Bring to a boil over high heat; reduce heat and simmer until potatoes are nearly tender, about 15 minutes. Add the meatballs and the remaining cilantro; simmer for 30 minutes. Season to taste with salt and black pepper.

Homemade Biscuit Mix

Ingredients

10 cups all-purpose flour
1/2 cup baking powder
2 tablespoons white sugar
2 teaspoons salt
1 1/4 cups vegetable oil

Directions

Combine flour, baking powder, sugar and salt in a mixing bowl. Add oil and mix with a fork or pastry blender; you should have small lumps throughout the mixture.

Store in an airtight container in a cool, dry place for up to three months.

Homemade Manti (Traditional Turkish Dumplings)

Ingredients

2 cups flour
1/2 teaspoon salt
2 eggs
1/2 teaspoon water, or as needed
2 onions, peeled
1/2 pound ground beef
salt and pepper to taste
3 tablespoons vegetable oil
1 tablespoon red pepper flakes
1 tablespoon minced garlic
1 (8 ounce) container plain yogurt

Directions

Combine the flour and salt in a mixing bowl. Add the eggs and water, mixing well with your hands. Add more water, if needed, to form a soft dough. Cover and set aside for at least 30 minutes.

Shred the onions and place them in a colander or sieve set over a bowl; drain the juice and discard. Combine the onion, ground beef, salt, and pepper; mix the meat well with a spoon until mashed.

Divide the dough into two portions and lightly flour a work surface. Keep one piece of dough covered while you roll out the second portion into a rectangle, rolling the dough as thin as you can. Cut the rectangle into 2-inch squares with a knife or pastry wheel.

Place about 2 teaspoons of the meat filling in the center of each square. Seal the dumplings by gathering the edges of the dough and pinching them together at the top to form a bundle. Transfer the finished manti to a floured plate, and sprinkle more flour over the manti to prevent sticking. Repeat with the second piece of dough.

Heat the oil and red pepper flakes in a small skillet over low heat just until the pepper flakes have started to color the oil; don't let them burn. Remove from the heat and keep warm. Stir the minced garlic into the yogurt and set aside.

Bring a large pot of salted water to a boil over medium-high heat, and cook the manti until the filling is no longer pink, and the dough is tender, 20 to 25 minutes. Drain well. Divide the manti among four plates. Spoon the yogurt sauce over the manti and drizzle each serving with the hot pepper oil.

Homemade Hash Browns

Ingredients

6 pounds medium potatoes
2 cups chopped green pepper
2 cups chopped sweet red pepper
1 large onion, chopped
1/2 cup butter or margarine
1 teaspoon salt
1 teaspoon pepper

Directions

Place potatoes in a Dutch oven and cover with water. Bring to a boil; cover and simmer for 15-20 minutes or until potatoes are tender but still firm. Cool slightly; peel and shred. In a Dutch oven, saute the peppers and onion in butter. Add the shredded potatoes; sprinkle with salt and pepper. Cook until golden brown.

Speedy Homemade Salsa

Ingredients

1 (14.5 ounce) can whole peeled tomatoes, drained
1/4 cup chopped red onion
1/4 cup chopped onion
1 jalapeno pepper, seeded
1 tablespoon cider vinegar
1 tablespoon minced fresh cilantro
1 clove garlic, peeled
1 teaspoon ground cumin
1/4 teaspoon salt

Directions

In a food processor, combine all ingredients; cover and process until chunky. Transfer to a small bowl.

Homemade Maple Syrup

Ingredients

1 cup water
1 cup white sugar
1 cup brown sugar
1 tablespoon maple flavored extract

Directions

Bring the water, white sugar, and brown sugar to a boil in a saucepan over medium-high heat. Reduce heat to medium-low, and stir in the maple extract; simmer 3 minutes longer.

Homemade Egg Noodles

Ingredients

2 cups all-purpose flour
1/4 teaspoon salt
1/4 teaspoon baking powder
4 egg yolks

Directions

Sift together the flour, salt and baking powder. Add egg yolks and mix until dry ingredients are moistened.

Press into a ball and cut in quarters. Roll out on floured surface 1/8 to 1/4 inch thick; cut to desired width and length. Lay on linen dish towel or wooden dowel to dry.

Add to broth such as chicken or turkey and cook until done.

Homemade Horseradish

Ingredients

1 cup peeled and cubed
horseradish root
3/4 cup white vinegar
2 teaspoons white sugar
1/4 teaspoon salt

Directions

In an electric food processor or blender, process horseradish root, vinegar, sugar and salt. Carefully remove the cover of the processor or blender, keeping your face away from the container. Cover and store the horseradish in the refrigerator.

Jean's Homemade Chicken Noodle Soup

Ingredients

2 (14 ounce) cans chicken broth
2 cups water
3 carrots, chopped
3 stalks celery, chopped
1 pinch ground black pepper
3 slices fresh ginger root
1 tablespoon vegetable oil
1/2 cup chopped cooked chicken breast meat
1/2 cup egg noodles

Directions

In a large pot over medium heat combine the broth, water, carrots, celery and ground black pepper and allow to cook. In a medium skillet over medium high heat, combine the ginger, oil and chicken. Saute for about 5 minutes and remove the sliced ginger.

Add the chicken to the broth mixture, bring to a boil and then add the egg noodles. Continue to cook over medium heat for about 15 minutes until noodles and vegetables are tender.

Homemade Spaghetti Sauce

Ingredients

1 chopped onion
5 cloves garlic, chopped
2 teaspoons olive oil
2 (28 ounce) cans peeled ground tomatoes in paste
1 (6 ounce) can Italian-style tomato paste
7 cups water
3 tablespoons Italian seasoning
2 tablespoons dried basil
1 teaspoon white sugar
1/2 cup red wine
1 pinch crushed red pepper

Directions

In large saucepan over medium heat, saute onion and garlic in olive oil until soft. Stir in tomatoes, tomato paste, water, Italian seasoning, basil, sugar, wine, and crushed red pepper. Reduce heat to low and simmer 3 hours, stirring occasionally. Serve.

Homemade Ginger Ale

Ingredients

1 1/2 tablespoons grated fresh ginger root
1 cup sugar
1/4 teaspoon active dry yeast
1 lemon, juiced
water

Directions

Into an empty 2-liter soda bottle, put the ginger root, sugar, yeast, and lemon juice. Fill the rest of the way with water. Screw the cap onto the bottle as tight as possible. Shake the bottle well, then leave at room temperature until the bottle is too hard to squeeze, about 2 days. Refrigerate. To serve, pour through a tea strainer.

Homemade Dog Food

Ingredients

6 cups water
1 pound ground turkey
2 cups brown rice
1 teaspoon dried rosemary
1/2 (16 ounce) package frozen broccoli, carrots and cauliflower combination

Directions

Place the water, ground turkey, rice, and rosemary into a large Dutch oven. Stir until the ground turkey is broken up and evenly distributed throughout the mixture; bring to a boil over high heat, then reduce heat to low and simmer for 20 minutes. Add the frozen vegetables, and cook for an additional 5 minutes. Remove from heat and cool. Refrigerate until using.

Buddy's and Bubba's Homemade Dog Food

Ingredients

2 chicken leg quarters
1 cup brown rice
1 pound ground beef
2/3 cup rolled oats
1 (10 ounce) package chopped frozen spinach, thawed and squeezed dry
2 cups frozen chopped broccoli, thawed
1 (15 ounce) can kidney beans - rinsed, drained and mashed
2 carrots, shredded
1 clove garlic, minced (optional)
1 cup cottage cheese
1/2 cup olive oil

Directions

Place the chicken leg quarters in a large pot, and fill with enough water to cover by 1 inch. Bring to a boil, then reduce heat to medium-low, cover, and simmer 40 minutes. Remove the legs and allow to cool. Strain and return the cooking liquid to the pot. Once the legs have cooled. remove and discard the skin and bones; chop the meat, and set aside.

Stir the brown rice into the reserved chicken broth and bring to a boil. Reduce heat to medium-low, cover, and simmer until the rice is tender, 45 to 50 minutes. Drain off any excess liquid, and add the rice to the bowl with the chicken.

Heat a large skillet over medium-high heat, and add the ground beef. Cook and stir until the beef is crumbly and no longer pink, about 7 minutes. Pour off any excess grease, and place the beef into the bowl. Stir in the oats, spinach, broccoli, kidney beans, carrots, garlic, cottage cheese, and olive oil. Store the dog food in resealable containers in the freezer. Thaw the daily portions overnight in the refrigerator.

Homemade Shake and Bake Mixture

Ingredients

4 cups dry bread crumbs
1/3 cup vegetable oil
1 tablespoon salt
1 tablespoon paprika
1 tablespoon celery salt
1 teaspoon ground black pepper
1/2 teaspoon garlic salt
1/2 teaspoon minced garlic
1/4 teaspoon minced onion
1 pinch dried basil leaves
1 pinch dried parsley
1 pinch dried oregano

Directions

In a large resealable plastic bag combine the crumbs, oil, salt, paprika, celery salt, pepper, garlic salt, minced garlic, minced onion, basil, parsley and oregano. Seal bag and shake all ingredients together.

Homemade Four Cheese Ravioli

Ingredients

Ravioli Dough:
2 cups all-purpose flour
1 pinch salt
1 teaspoon olive oil
2 eggs
1 1/2 tablespoons water

Ravioli Filling:
1 (8 ounce) container ricotta cheese
1 (4 ounce) package cream cheese, softened
1/2 cup shredded mozzarella cheese
1/2 cup provolone cheese, shredded
1 egg
1 1/2 teaspoons dried parsley

Pesto-Alfredo Cream Sauce:
2 tablespoons olive oil
2 cloves garlic, crushed
3 tablespoons prepared basil pesto sauce
2 cups heavy cream
1/4 cup grated Parmesan cheese
1 (24 ounce) jar marinara sauce

Egg Wash:
1 egg
1 tablespoon water

Directions

Mound the flour and salt together on a work surface and form a well. Beat the teaspoon of olive oil, 2 eggs, and water in a bowl. Pour half the egg mixture into the well. Begin mixing the egg with the flour with one hand; use your other hand to keep the flour mound steady. Add the remaining egg mixture and knead to form a dough.

Knead the dough until smooth, 8 to 10 minutes; add more flour if the dough is too sticky. Form the dough into a ball and wrap tightly with plastic. Refrigerate for 1 hour.

While the dough is resting, prepare the ravioli filling. Combine the ricotta cheese, cream cheese, mozzarella cheese, provolone cheese, egg, and parsley and mix well. Set the filling aside.

Heat 2 tablespoons of olive oil in a skillet over medium heat. Add the crushed garlic and pesto sauce and cook for one minute. Pour in the heavy cream, raise the heat to high, and bring the sauce to a boil. Reduce the heat and simmer for 5 minutes. Add the Parmesan cheese and stir until the cheese melts. Remove the pan from the heat and keep warm.

Meanwhile, in a separate saucepan, warm the marinara sauce over medium-low heat.

Preheat an oven to 375 degrees F (190 degrees C). Beat the egg with the tablespoon of water to make the egg wash.

Roll out the pasta dough into thin sheets no thicker than a nickel. To assemble the ravioli, brush the egg wash over a sheet of pasta. Drop the filling mixture on the dough by teaspoonfuls about one inch apart. Cover the filling with the top sheet of pasta, pressing out the air from around each portion of filling. Press firmly around the filling to seal. Cut into individual ravioli with a knife or pizza cutter. Seal the edges.

Fill a large pot with lightly salted water and bring to a rolling boil over high heat. Stir in the ravioli, and return to a boil. Cook uncovered, stirring occasionally, until the ravioli float to the top and the filling is hot, 4 to 8 minutes. Drain well.

Grease a baking sheet. Place the cooked ravioli on the sheet pan and bake in the preheated oven until brown, about 4 minutes.

Homemade Potater Tots

Ingredients

2 russet potatoes
1/4 cup chopped fresh chives
(optional)
2 teaspoons salt
1 teaspoon white pepper
vegetable oil for frying

Directions

Place the potatoes in a saucepan of water to cover, and bring to a boil over medium heat. Reduce heat, and simmer until the potatoes are cooked through but still firm, about 20 minutes. Remove from the water, and peel the cooked potatoes while still hot.

Line a baking sheet with parchment paper and set aside.

Shred the potatoes with a box grater, and place the shredded potatoes in a bowl. Lightly mix in the chives, salt, and white pepper. Spoon the potato mixture into a piping bag with a 1/2-inch round tip.

Pipe the potato mixture onto the parchment paper in a long, 1/2-inch wide rope. Place the baking sheet into the refrigerator until the potato mixture has cooled and set, about 1 hour. Cut the potato strip into 1-inch lengths.

Heat vegetable oil in a deep-fryer or large saucepan to 350 degrees F (175 degrees C). Working in batches, deep-fry the potato pieces until crisp and golden brown.

Homemade Barbecue Sauce

Ingredients

2 tablespoons butter, melted
2 tablespoons chopped onion
1 tablespoon chopped green bell pepper
1 cup water
1 cup ketchup
2 teaspoons mustard powder
1 teaspoon salt
1 teaspoon celery seed
2 tablespoons brown sugar
2 teaspoons lemon juice

Directions

In a medium nonporous bowl, combine the butter or margarine, onion, green bell pepper, water, ketchup, mustard powder, salt, celery seed, brown sugar and lemon juice. Mix well and use on your choice of meat.

Homemade Yummy Fudge

Ingredients

6 ounces cream cheese, softened
1/8 teaspoon salt
1/2 teaspoon vanilla extract
4 cups confectioners' sugar, sifted
4 (1 ounce) squares unsweetened chocolate, melted and cooled
1 cup chopped walnuts

Directions

Line an 8x8 inch dish with foil.

In a medium bowl, beat cream cheese until smooth. Beat in salt and vanilla. Beat in confectioners' sugar, a little at a time, until smooth. Stir in melted chocolate. Fold in walnuts. Spread into prepared pan. Chill 1 hour, until firm. Cut into one inch squares.

Homemade Marshmallows II

Ingredients

3 cups white sugar
1/4 cup corn syrup
1/4 teaspoon salt
3/4 cup water
2 teaspoons vanilla extract
1 cup confectioners' sugar for dusting

Directions

Generously coat a 9x13 dish with cooking spray.

In a large saucepan, combine sugar, corn syrup, salt and water. Heat to between 234 and 240 degrees F (112 to 116 degrees C), or until a small amount of syrup dropped into cold water forms a soft ball that flattens when removed from the water and placed on a flat surface. Remove from heat and beat with an electric mixer until stiff peaks form, 10 to 12 minutes. Stir in vanilla. Pour into prepared pan.

Chill in refrigerator 8 hours or overnight. To cut, loosen edges with a knife. Dust surface with confectioners' sugar, and turn out onto a waxed paper lined surface. Dust with confectioners' sugar again and cut with a knife.

Homemade Apple Cider

Ingredients

10 apples, quartered
3/4 cup white sugar
1 tablespoon ground cinnamon
1 tablespoon ground allspice

Directions

Place apples in a large stockpot and add enough water cover by at least 2 inches. Stir in sugar, cinnamon, and allspice. Bring to a boil. Boil, uncovered, for 1 hour. Cover pot, reduce heat, and simmer for 2 hours.

Strain apple mixture though a fine mesh sieve. Discard solids. Drain cider again though a cheesecloth lined sieve. Refrigerate until cold.

Homemade Beef Breakfast Sausage Patties

Ingredients

1 tablespoon brown sugar
2 teaspoons dried sage
2 teaspoons salt
2 teaspoons dried basil
1 teaspoon ground black pepper
1 teaspoon onion powder
1/4 teaspoon dried marjoram
1/8 teaspoon crushed red pepper
flakes
2 pounds ground beef

Directions

Stir the brown sugar, sage, salt, basil, black pepper, onion powder, marjoram, and red pepper flakes together in a small bowl. Place the ground beef in a large bowl; mix the spice blend into the ground beef with your hands until evenly integrated. Refrigerate for 24 hours to let the flavors blend.

Divide the ground beef mixture into 8 patties.

Place a large skillet over medium heat; cook the patties in the skillet until firm, hot, and cooked in the center, 5 to 7 minutes per side. An instant-read thermometer inserted into the center should read 160 degrees F (70 degrees C).

Homemade Dog Biscuits

Ingredients

3 1/2 cups all-purpose flour
2 cups wheat bran
1 cup cornmeal
4 teaspoons salt
1 tablespoon garlic powder
2 cups whole wheat flour
1 cup rye flour
1/2 cup nonfat dry milk powder
2 1/4 teaspoons active dry yeast
1/4 cup warm water
2 cups tomato juice

Directions

Preheat oven to 300 degrees F (150 degrees C).

Dissolve the yeast in the warm water. Stir in the tomato juice.

Combine the all-purpose flour, bran, grits or cornmeal, salt, garlic powder, whole wheat flour, rye flour and non-fat dry milk powder. Stir in the yeast mixture. Dough should be very stiff.

On a lightly floured board roll dough out to 1/3 to 1/2 inch thick. Cut into desired size with a knife or cookie cutters. Place on ungreased cookie sheet.

Bake at 300 degrees F (150 degrees C) for 1 hour. Turn oven off and leave biscuits overnight or for at least 4 hours in oven to harden.

Homemade Creme Liqueur

Ingredients

1 (14 ounce) can sweetened
condensed milk
1 cup coffee-flavored liqueur
1 cup heavy whipping cream
4 eggs

Directions

Combine condensed milk, liqueur, cream, and eggs in a blender,
and whip until smooth. Serve over ice, if desired.

Homemade Chewy Granola Bars

Ingredients

1/2 cup packed brown sugar
1/3 cup peanut butter
1/4 cup corn syrup
1/4 cup butter, melted
1 teaspoon vanilla extract
1 1/2 cups quick-cooking oats
1/4 cup sunflower kernels
1/4 cup raisins
3 tablespoons toasted wheat germ
1 tablespoon sesame seeds
1/2 cup semisweet chocolate chips

Directions

In a small mixing bowl, combine the brown sugar, peanut butter, corn syrup, butter and vanilla. Stir in the oats, sunflower kernels, raisins, wheat germ and sesame seeds. Fold in chocolate chips.

Press into an 8-in. square baking dish coated with nonstick cooking spray. Bake at 350 degrees F for 15-20 minutes or until set and edges are browned. Cool completely on a wire rack. Cut into bars.

Easy Homemade Pizza

Ingredients

1 (12 inch) pre-baked pizza crust
1 (14 ounce) jar Ragu® Pizza
Sauce - Homemade Style
1 cup shredded mozzarella
cheese
Your Favorite Pizza Toppings
(sliced pepperoni, mushrooms,
bell peppers, pitted ripe olives,
onions), optional

Directions

Preheat oven to 350 degrees F. Arrange pizza crust on ungreased
cookie sheet. Spoon on Pizza Sauce, then sprinkle with cheese and
Toppings.

Bake 15 minutes or until cheese is melted.

Easy Homemade Vanilla Ice Cream

Ingredients

4 cups half-and-half or light cream
1 (14 ounce) can EAGLE BRAND®Sweetened Condensed Milk
2 tablespoons vanilla extract

Directions

In large bowl, combine ingredients; mix well. Pour into ice cream freezer container. Freeze according to manufacturer's instructions. Freeze leftovers.

Homemade Chocolate Sandwich Cookies

Ingredients

2 (18.25 ounce) packages devil's food cake mix
4 eggs
1 cup shortening

Directions

Preheat oven to 350 degrees F (180 degrees C).

Blend the above ingredients together with a pastry blender until mixed.

Roll in balls about the size of a quarter and place on ungreased baking sheets. Make an even number of balls.

Bake for 10 minutes. Let cookies stand on cookie sheet for 5-6 minutes before removing them to cooling rack. After cookies have cooled, put Cream Cheese Frosting (see recipe or use one can of pre-made frosting) between two cookies, putting bottom sides together.

NOTE: Adding chopped pecans to the cookies without making them into sandwiches is also very good. Spice cake mix can be used in place of Devil's food.

Creamy Homemade Chicken Stew

Ingredients

1 cup lowfat evaporated milk
1/4 cup all-purpose flour
1 1/2 pounds chicken leg meat
3/4 pound small fresh button mushrooms
2 potatoes, peeled and cubed
2 cups pearl onions
2 large carrots, coarsely chopped
2 1/4 cups frozen green peas, thawed
1 cup chicken broth
1/2 teaspoon salt
1/4 teaspoon ground black pepper
1/2 teaspoon dried marjoram
1/4 teaspoon dried rosemary
1/4 cup chopped fresh parsley

Directions

In a small bowl stir together evaporated milk and flour until smooth. Place chicken, mushrooms, potatoes, onions, carrots and peas in slow cooker. Pour in milk mixture and broth. Season with salt, pepper, marjoram and rosemary. Cook on low 6 hours. Stir in parsley just before serving.

Homemade Angel Food Cake

Ingredients

18 egg whites
2 teaspoons cream of tartar
1 pinch salt
1 1/2 cups white sugar
1 cup cake flour
1/2 cup confectioners' sugar
1 teaspoon vanilla extract

Directions

Preheat oven to 350 degrees F (175 degrees C). Sift cake flour and confectioners sugar together 5 times and set aside.

In a large clean bowl, whip egg whites with a pinch of salt until foamy. Add cream of tartar and continue beating until soft peaks form. Gradually add sugar while beating, and continue to beat until very stiff. Add vanilla.

Quickly fold in flour mixture. Pour into a 10 inch tube pan.

Bake at 350 degrees F (175 degrees C) for 45 minutes.

Homemade Pancake Mix

Ingredients

4 cups all-purpose flour
2 cups whole wheat flour
2/3 cup sugar
2 tablespoons baking powder
1 tablespoon baking soda
ADDITIONAL INGREDIENTS FOR
PANCAKES:
1 egg
3/4 cup milk
ADDITIONAL INGREDIENTS FOR
BLUEBERRY BANANA
PANCAKES:
1 egg
3/4 cup milk
1 medium ripe banana, mashed
3/4 cup blueberries

Directions

In a bowl, combine the first five ingredients. Store in an airtight container in a cool dry place for up to 6 months.

To prepare pancakes: In a bowl, combine egg and milk. Whisk in 1 cup pancake mix. Pour batter by 1/4 cupfuls onto a lightly greased hot griddle; turn when bubbles form on top of pancakes. Cook until second side is golden brown

To prepare blueberry banana pancakes: In a bowl, combine egg, milk and banana. Whisk in 1 cup pancake mix. Fold in blueberries. Cook as directed above.

My Momma's Easy Homemade Veggie Soup

Ingredients

3 pounds ground beef
6 potatoes, peeled and cubed
water to cover
4 (15 ounce) cans mixed
vegetables, drained
1 onion, chopped
2 cups chopped cabbage
1 (15 ounce) can tomato sauce
2 tablespoons ground black
pepper
salt to taste

Directions

Place the ground beef in a large skillet over medium high heat.
Saute for 10 to 15 minutes, or until browned and crumbly; set aside.

In a large pot over high heat, combine the potatoes with water to
cover and cook for 20 minutes, or until potatoes are almost tender.

Add the mixed vegetables, onion, cabbage, tomato sauce, reserved
ground beef and ground black pepper.

Bring to a boil, reduce heat to low and simmer for 1 1/2 to 2 hours.
Season with salt to taste.

Real Homemade Tamales

Ingredients

Tamale Filling:
1 1/4 pounds pork loin
1 large onion, halved
1 clove garlic
4 dried California chile pods
2 cups water
1 1/2 teaspoons salt

Tamale Dough:
2 cups masa harina
1 (10.5 ounce) can beef broth
1 teaspoon baking powder
1/2 teaspoon salt
2/3 cup lard
1 (8 ounce) package dried corn husks
1 cup sour cream

Directions

Place pork into a Dutch oven with onion and garlic, and add water to cover. Bring to a boil, then reduce heat to low and simmer until the meat is cooked through, about 2 hours.

Use rubber gloves to remove stems and seeds from the chile pods. Place chiles in a saucepan with 2 cups of water. Simmer, uncovered, for 20 minutes, then remove from heat to cool. Transfer the chiles and water to a blender and blend until smooth. Strain the mixture, stir in salt, and set aside. Shred the cooked meat and mix in one cup of the chile sauce.

Soak the corn husks in a bowl of warm water. In a large bowl, beat the lard with a tablespoon of the broth until fluffy. Combine the masa harina, baking powder and salt; stir into the lard mixture, adding more broth as necessary to form a spongy dough.

Spread the dough out over the corn husks to 1/4 to 1/2 inch thickness. Place one tablespoon of the meat filling into the center. Fold the sides of the husks in toward the center and place in a steamer. Steam for 1 hour.

Remove tamales from husks and drizzle remaining chile sauce over. Top with sour cream. For a creamy sauce, mix sour cream into the chile sauce.

CPSIA information can be obtained
at www.ICGtesting.com
Printed in the USA
BVHW011551270421
605947BV00013B/2469